Satisfying Low Carb Diet

920 Essential Low Carb Cookbook + 2500 Days Easy, Delicious Recipes to Start Losing Weight.

CATHERINE RICE

ISBN: 9798327854765

Imprint: Independently published

Cover design by: Art Painter

Library of Congress Control Number: 2018675309

Printed in the United States of America

DEDICATION

To all the brave souls embarking on a journey toward a healthier, happier life.

This book is dedicated to you, the seekers of balance, vitality, and well-being. May these recipes inspire you to nourish your body, delight your senses, and find joy in every meal.

To my family and friends, whose unwavering support and encouragement made this book possible. Your love and belief in me have been my greatest strength.

And to the pioneers of low-carb living, whose knowledge and passion continue to light the way for so many. Your dedication to wellness has touched countless lives.

May this book be a beacon of inspiration, guiding you toward your best self?

Table of Contents

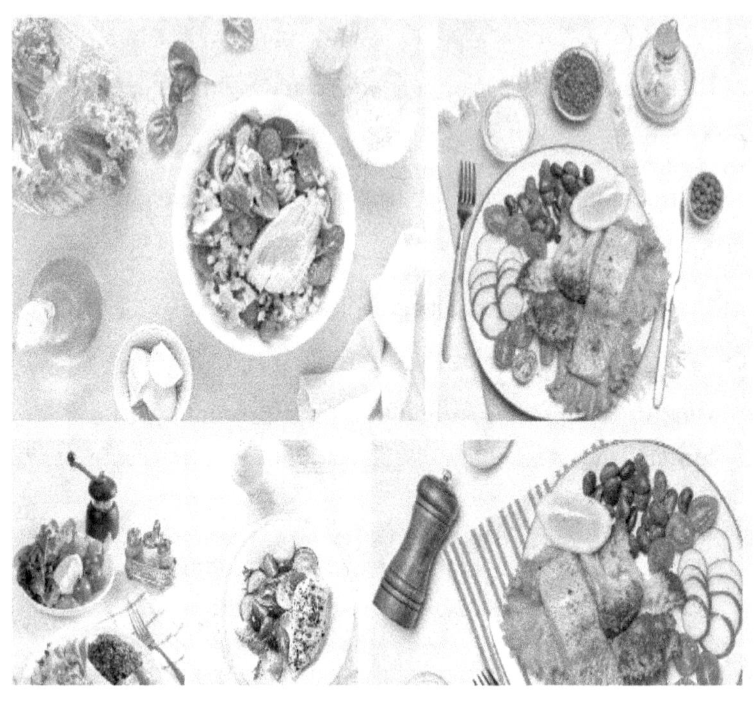

INTRODUCTION

The low-carb diet has been shown to be effective in reducing body weight, presenting an advantage over other methods in numerous scientific studies

It is an adaptation of low-carbohydrate diets that has been used since 1920.

The great advantage of the method is the fact that, even if there is a restriction on carbohydrates, it does not involve counting calories, that is, it is the quality, the type of food that must be controlled and not the quantity.

Do you want to eat real food (as much as you want) and improve your health and weight? It may sound "too good to be true", but LCHF (low carb, high fat) is a method that has been used for 150 years. Now, modern science backs it up with proof that it works.

No need to weigh your food, no counting calories, no bizarre "meal replacements," no medication. There is only real food and common sense.

CHAPTER 1

Low-carb diets: Discover the most popular

With so many diet options currently available, it can be difficult to understand what each one offers and which one best fits the body, routine and well-being of those who want to lose weight.

Of the dietary programs most sought after by those who want to lose weight today, low- carb diets are certainly among the most sought after.

This methodology became famous for proposing a reduced consumption of carbohydrates to reduce the weight of the scale, and the three best-known plans are the low carb diet , the ketogenic diet (keto) and the Paleolithic diet.

Less refined carbohydrates, more real food: this is the proposal followed by low-carb diets. However, each one has its own particularities, benefits and caveats.

Find out more about the three most popular low-carb diets and choose the one that best suits you and your goals:

How it works?

To give you an idea, the guideline in a conventional diet is that 50 to 55% of what is eaten per day is carbohydrates. In low carb methods, the macronutrient can make up between 45% and 5% of what is consumed daily.

Drastically reducing carbohydrate intake is one of the most classic strategies for losing weight, and the reason for this negligible carbohydrate intake is to control insulin.

"When we consume foods rich in carbohydrates, there is an increase in glucose and basal insulin, which can lead to a robust reserve of the nutrient and, consequently, an increase in body fat. When consuming less carbohydrates, insulin production decreases, leading to weight loss", explains Gabriela Cilla, clinical, sports and functional nutritionist, from São Paulo.

The program lasts a minimum of three weeks and can last up to six months, thus repeat the satisfying low-carb meals. Generally, because of the restriction, some nutritionists recommend a 40-day diet. Everything will depend on the professional and the needs and limitations of each individual.

Released foods

• Meat, fish and eggs

• Beef, lamb, chicken (thigh and drumstick), seafood, shrimp, salmon, trout, sardines and eggs.

• Fat and oil

• Ghee (clarified butter), butter, extra virgin olive oil and coconut oil.

• Nuts and seeds

• Almond, peanut, walnut, coconut and chia seeds, flaxseed, pumpkin and sunflower.

• Herbs and spices

• Salt (little!), herbs and spices (pepper, garlic, ginger, cinnamon, cardamom, thyme, oregano and sage).

Although it seems like a healthy idea, some fruits are notorious villains in this diet because they have high levels of carbohydrates. A medium apple, for example, has 20 to 25 grams of carbohydrates which for many may be the recommended dose for the entire day.

To avoid falling for this trick and compromising weight loss, we have listed five fruits with a low amount of carbohydrates that can be enjoyed by those who follow a low-carb diet. Check out:

Avocado

One of today's favorite fruits, avocado is rich in healthy monounsaturated fats, vitamins, minerals and fiber, but is low in carbohydrates. A whole avocado has just two grams of carbohydrates, making it an approved food for this style of diet.

Blackberry

One cup of blackberries has six grams of carbohydrates, which fits into the diet. Furthermore, the fruit is rich in fiber which, when in contact with the stomach, makes you feel fuller, less likely to want to eat and also reduces the intake of sugar and fat into the body.

Coconut

Half a cup of the fruit has 13 grams of healthy fat and about 2.5 grams of carbohydrates. However, when purchasing dehydrated or flaked coconut, make sure that no extra sugar has been added.

Lemon

Citrus fruit can be used as juice, tea or seasoning, as half a serving of a lemon has less than ½ gram of carbohydrates, just two calories, as well as vitamin C and calcium.

Strawberry

A full cup of strawberries has eight grams of carbohydrates, and the best part about this fruit is its versatility: add it to Greek yogurt, add it to a salad, throw it in water for flavor, or even use the strawberry as the base of a low carb dessert.

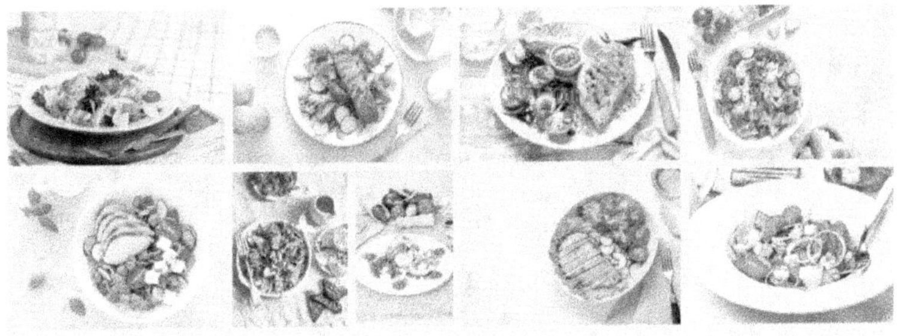

CHAPTER 2

Satisfying low-carb meal that supports your health and dietary goals

Breakfast Recipes
1. **Keto Pancakes**

Ingredients:

2 eggs, 1/4 cup almond flour, 1/4 cup cream cheese, 1/2 tsp baking powder, a pinch of salt.

Instructions:

Blend all ingredients. Cook on a greased skillet over medium heat until golden brown.

2. <u>Chia Seed Pudding</u>

Ingredients:

2 tbsp chia seeds, 1 cup unsweetened almond milk, 1 tsp vanilla extract, a pinch of stevia (optional).

Instructions:

Mix all ingredients in a bowl. Refrigerate overnight.

3. <u>Greek Yogurt with Berries</u>

Ingredients:

1 cup Greek yogurt, 1/2 cup mixed berries, 1 tbsp chopped nuts.

Instructions:

Combine all ingredients in a bowl and enjoy.

4. <u>Egg Muffins</u>

Ingredients:

6 eggs, 1/2 cup diced bell peppers, 1/2 cup spinach, 1/4 cup shredded cheese, salt, and pepper.

Instructions:

Mix all ingredients, pour into a greased muffin tin, and bake at 350°F for 20 minutes.

5. Cottage Cheese with Flaxseeds

Ingredients:

1 cup cottage cheese, 1 tbsp flaxseeds, a pinch of cinnamon.

Instructions:

Mix all ingredients in a bowl.

6. Avocado Smoothie

Ingredients:

1/2 avocado, 1 cup spinach, 1/2 cup unsweetened almond milk, 1 tbsp chia seeds.

Instructions:

Blend all ingredients until smooth.

7. <u>Scrambled Eggs with Spinach and Feta</u>

Ingredients:

2 eggs, 1 cup spinach, 1/4 cup feta cheese, salt, and pepper.

Instructions:

Sauté spinach, add beaten eggs, and cook until done. Sprinkle with feta cheese.

8. <u>Keto Oatmeal</u>

Ingredients:

2 tbsp flaxseed meal, 2 tbsp chia seeds, 1/2 cup unsweetened almond milk, 1 tsp vanilla extract.

Instructions:

Mix all ingredients and heat in a microwave or on the stove until thickened.

9. <u>Bacon and Egg Cups</u>

Ingredients:

6 bacon slices, 6 eggs, salt, and pepper.

Instructions:

Line a muffin tin with bacon slices, crack an egg into each, and bake at 350°F for 15-20 minutes.

10. <u>Salmon and Cream Cheese Omelet</u>

Ingredients:

2 eggs, 1/4 cup smoked salmon, 2 tbsp cream cheese, salt, and pepper.

Instructions:

Make an omelet with all ingredients in a greased skillet.

Lunch Recipes

1. <u>Chicken Caesar Salad</u>

Ingredients:

1 grilled chicken breast, 2 cups romaine lettuce, 2 tbsp Parmesan cheese, 2 tbsp Caesar dressing.

Instructions:

Combine all ingredients in a bowl.

2. <u>Turkey Lettuce Wraps</u>

Ingredients:

4 large lettuce leaves, 4 slices turkey breast, 1/2 avocado, 1/2 bell pepper, sliced.

<u>Instructions:</u>

Wrap turkey, avocado, and bell pepper in lettuce leaves.

3. <u>Tuna Salad</u>

Ingredients:

1 can tuna, 2 tbsp mayonnaise, 1/4 cup diced celery, salt, and pepper.

Instructions:

Mix all ingredients in a bowl.

4. <u>Greek Salad</u>

Ingredients:

1 cup cherry tomatoes, 1/2 cucumber, 1/4 cup red onion, 1/4 cup Kalamata olives, 1/4 cup feta cheese, olive oil, lemon juice.

Instructions:

Combine all ingredients and toss with olive oil and lemon juice.

5. <u>Egg Salad</u>

Ingredients:

4 hard-boiled eggs, 2 tbsp mayonnaise, 1 tsp mustard, salt, and pepper.

Instructions:

Chop eggs and mix with mayonnaise, mustard, salt, and pepper.

6. Avocado Chicken Salad

Ingredients:

1 grilled chicken breast, 1/2 avocado, 1 tbsp olive oil, lemon juice, salt, and pepper.

Instructions:

Dice chicken and avocado, and mix with olive oil, lemon juice, salt, and pepper.

7. Stuffed Bell Peppers

Ingredients:

2 bell peppers, 1/2 lb ground beef, 1/2 cup diced tomatoes, 1/4 cup shredded cheese.

Instructions:

Cut tops off bell peppers, stuff with beef and tomatoes, and bake at 375°F for 20 minutes. Sprinkle with cheese.

8. <u>Cobb Salad</u>

Ingredients:

2 cups mixed greens, 1 boiled egg, 1/2 avocado, 1/2 cup cooked chicken, 2 tbsp blue cheese, 2 slices bacon, crumbled.

Instructions:

Combine all ingredients in a bowl.

9. <u>Zucchini Boats</u>

Ingredients:

2 zucchinis, 1/2 lb ground turkey, 1/2 cup marinara sauce, 1/4 cup shredded mozzarella.

Instructions:

Hollow out zucchinis, stuff with turkey and marinara sauce, and bake at 375°F for 20 minutes. Top with cheese.

10. <u>Shrimp Avocado Salad</u>

Ingredients:

1 cup cooked shrimp, 1/2 avocado, 1/4 cup diced cucumber, 1 tbsp olive oil, lemon juice.

Instructions:

Combine all ingredients in a bowl.

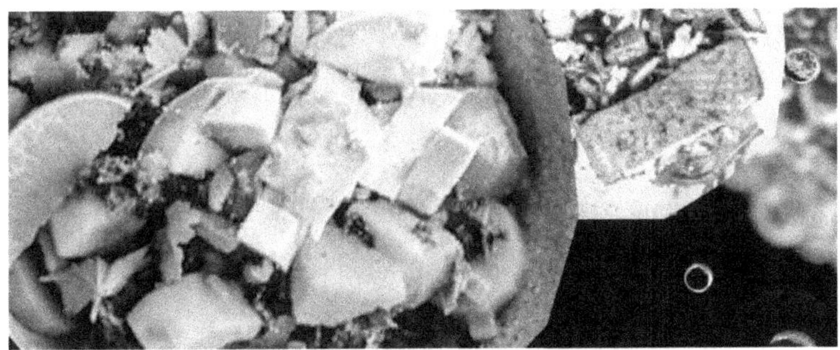

Dinner Recipes

1. <u>Grilled Steak with Asparagus</u>

Ingredients:

1 steak, 1 bunch asparagus, olive oil, salt, and pepper.

Instructions:

Season steak and grill. Toss asparagus with olive oil, salt, and pepper, and grill until tender.

2. <u>Lemon Garlic Shrimp</u>

Ingredients:

1 lb shrimp, 2 tbsp olive oil, 3 garlic cloves, minced, lemon juice, salt, and pepper.

Instructions:

Sauté garlic in olive oil, add shrimp and lemon juice, and cook until shrimp is done.

3. <u>Cauliflower Pizza</u>

Ingredients:

1 head cauliflower, 1/2 cup mozzarella, 1 egg, 1/2 cup marinara sauce, toppings of choice.

Instructions:

Pulse cauliflower into rice, mix with mozzarella and egg, bake at 400°F for 15 minutes. Add toppings and bake for another 10 minutes.

4. <u>Beef and Broccoli Stir-Fry</u>

Ingredients:

1 lb beef strips, 2 cups broccoli florets, 2 tbsp soy sauce, 1 tbsp sesame oil, garlic, and ginger.

Instructions:

Sauté garlic and ginger in sesame oil, add beef and cook. Add broccoli and soy sauce, and cook until tender.

5. <u>Pork Chops with Green Beans</u>

Ingredients:

2 pork chops, 1 lb green beans, olive oil, salt, and pepper.

Instructions:

Season pork chops and grill. Toss green beans with olive oil, salt, and pepper, and roast at 400°F for 20 minutes.

6. <u>Zoodle Alfredo</u>

Ingredients:

2 zucchinis, 1/2 cup heavy cream, 1/4 cup Parmesan cheese, 1 garlic clove, minced.

Instructions:

Spiralize zucchinis, cook garlic in heavy cream, add Parmesan, and toss with zoodles.

7. <u>Baked Cod with Lemon Butter</u>

Ingredients:

2 cod fillets, 2 tbsp butter, lemon juice, salt, and pepper.

Instructions:

Season cod, top with butter and lemon juice, and bake at 375°F for 20 minutes.

8. Chicken Fajitas

Ingredients:

2 chicken breasts, 1 bell pepper, 1 onion, 2 tbsp olive oil, fajita seasoning.

Instructions:

Slice chicken and vegetables, toss with olive oil and seasoning, and cook in a skillet until done.

9. Eggplant Parmesan

Ingredients:

 1 eggplant, 1/2 cup marinara sauce, 1/2 cup mozzarella, olive oil, salt, and pepper.

Instructions:

Slice and roast eggplant, top with marinara and mozzarella, and bake at 375°F for 20 minutes.

10. Garlic Butter Mushrooms

Ingredients:

1 lb mushrooms, 2 tbsp butter, 3 garlic cloves, minced, parsley.

Instructions:

Sauté garlic in butter, adds mushrooms, and cook until tender. Sprinkle with parsley.

Snack Recipes

1. Guacamole with Veggie Sticks

Ingredients:

2 avocados, 1/4 cup diced onion, 1/4 cup diced tomato, lime juice, salt, and pepper.

Instructions:

Mash avocados and mix with onion, tomato, lime juice, salt, and pepper. Serve with veggie sticks.

2. Cheese Crisps

Ingredients:

1 cup shredded cheese.

Instructions:

Place small mounds of cheese on a parchment-lined baking sheet and bake at 400°F for 5-7 minutes until crispy.

3. <u>Almond Butter Celery Sticks</u>

Ingredients:

3 celery sticks, 2 tbsp almond butter.

Instructions:

Spread almond butter on celery sticks.

4. <u>Keto Fat Bombs</u>

Ingredients:

1/2 cup coconut oil, 1/4 cup almond butter, 1/4 cup unsweetened cocoa powder, stevia to taste.

Instructions:

Melt coconut oil and almond butter, mix with cocoa powder and stevia, and pour into molds. Freeze until solid.

5. <u>Hard-Boiled Eggs</u>

Ingredients: 6 eggs.

Instructions:

Boil eggs for 10-12 minutes, cool, and peel.

6. <u>**Turkey Roll-Ups**</u>

Ingredients:

4 slices turkey breast, 4 slices cheese, 4 cucumber sticks.

Instructions:

Roll turkey and cheese around cucumber sticks.

7. <u>**Olives and Cheese**</u>

Ingredients:

1/2 cup olives, 1/4 cup cubed cheese.

Instructions:

Combine olives and cheese in a bowl.

8. <u>**Deviled Eggs**</u>

Ingredients:

6 hard-boiled eggs, 2 tbsp mayonnaise, 1 tsp mustard, salt, and pepper.

Instructions:

Halve eggs, mix yolks with mayonnaise and mustard, and spoon back into egg whites.

9. <u>Stuffed Mini Peppers</u>

Ingredients:

6 mini bell peppers, 1/4 cup cream cheese, herbs of choice.

Instructions:

Halve and deseed peppers, stuff with cream cheese mixed with herbs.

10. <u>Salami and Cheese</u>

Ingredients:

8 slices salami, 8 slices cheese.

Instructions:

Roll cheese in salami slices.

Dessert Recipes

1. <u>Chocolate Avocado Mousse</u>

Ingredients:

2 avocados, 1/4 cup unsweetened cocoa powder, 1/4 cup stevia or low-carb sweetener, 1 tsp vanilla extract.

Instructions:

Blend all ingredients until smooth.

2. <u>Berries and Cream</u>

Ingredients:

1/2 cup mixed berries, 1/4 cup whipped cream.

Instructions:

Top berries with whipped cream.

3. <u>Coconut Macaroons</u>

Ingredients:

2 cups shredded coconut, 1/4 cup almond flour, 1/4 cup stevia or low-carb sweetener, 2 egg whites.

Instructions:

Mix all ingredients, form into balls, and bake at 350°F for 15 minutes.

4. Keto Cheesecake Bites

Ingredients:

1 cup cream cheese, 1/4 cup stevia or low-carb sweetener, 1/2 tsp vanilla extract.

Instructions:

Mix all ingredients, form into balls, and refrigerate until firm.

5. Peanut Butter Cookies

Ingredients:

1 cup peanut butter, 1/2 cup stevia or low-carb sweetener, 1 egg.

Instructions:

Mix all ingredients, form into balls, press with a fork, and bake at 350°F for 10 minutes.

6. Almond Flour Brownies

Ingredients:

1 cup almond flour, 1/4 cup unsweetened cocoa powder, 1/2 cup stevia or low-carb sweetener, 2 eggs, 1/4 cup butter, melted.

Instructions:

Mix all ingredients, pour into a baking dish, and bake at 350°F for 20-25 minutes.

7. <u>Coconut Milk Popsicles</u>

Ingredients:

1 can coconut milk, 1/4 cup stevia or low-carb sweetener, 1 tsp vanilla extract.

Instructions:

Mix all ingredients, pour into molds, and freeze until solid.

8. <u>Lemon Bars</u>

Ingredients:

1 cup almond flour, 1/4 cup butter, 1/4 cup stevia or low-carb sweetener, 2 eggs, 1/2 cup lemon juice.

Instructions:

Mix almond flour and butter, press into a baking dish, bake at 350°F for 10 minutes. Mix remaining ingredients, pour over crust, and bake for another 15 minutes.

9. <u>Keto Chocolate Chip Cookies</u>

Ingredients:

1 cup almond flour, 1/4 cup butter, melted, 1/4 cup stevia or low-carb sweetener, 1 egg, 1/4 cup sugar-free chocolate chips.

Instructions:

 Mix all ingredients, form into balls, and bake at 350°F for 10-12 minutes.

10. <u>Cinnamon Almonds</u>

Ingredients:

2 cups almonds, 1/4 cup stevia or low-carb sweetener, 1 tsp cinnamon, 1 egg white.

Instructions:

Mix all ingredients, spread on a baking sheet, and bake at 300°F for 25 minutes, stirring occasionally.

CHAPTER 2

Light beer and wine are low in carbohydrates, while pure forms of drinks such as rum, whiskey, gin and vodka are free of the nutrient. However, excessive alcohol intake can slow down fat burning and cause weight gain, meaning the diet may not have the desired effect.

What is not allowed?

Skimmed milk

The weak point is that it has no fat.

Candy

They have sugar to give and sell.

Pastas

Retire pasta, lasagna, gnocchi…

Industrialized

They are not considered real food.

Corn

In any recipe, it is vetoed.

Breads

It is the ultimate symbol of carbohydrate.

Fruit juices

You have to avoid natural ones and nectar.

Tapioca

It's quite similar to bread.

Refrigerator

A real sugar pit.

Fruits with a high glycemic index

Banana, watermelon, mango, grape and pineapple are **examples.**

Rice

Neither white nor whole grain should be on the plate.

English potato

It has less fiber than other tubers.

Menu suggestion for those who want to start a low carb diet

DAY 1 (60% CARBOHYDRATE)

Breakfast:

1 Cup. (Tea) of coffee or tea as much as you like* + 2 eggs scrambled with pepper and turmeric + 2 medium slices of boiled sweet potato.

Morning snack:

1 banana mashed with 1 tbsp. (soup) of oat bran and 2 tbsp. chia (tea) + 1 cup. of ginger, cinnamon and clove tea .

Lunch:

Salad (mix of leaves, cherry tomatoes and sunflower seeds)

3 col. brown rice (soup)

2 col. (bean soup

1 medium grilled chicken fillet

4 col. cooked okra (soup)

Afternoon snack:

1 tangerine + 2 Brazil nuts + wrap: (sheet bread with 2 tablespoons of tuna, cottage cheese, grated carrot and lettuce).

To have lunch:

1 stick of whole meal spaghetti with Bolognese sauce (lean ground meat).

Supper:

3 small cookies with fiber + 1 cup. Of hibiscus tea.

DAY 2 (50% CARBOHYDRATE)

Breakfast:

1 glass (200 ml) of vegetable milk beaten with 1 prune and 1 tbsp. chia (soup) (mix 15 minutes beforehand).

Morning snack:

1 slice of whole meal bread with hummus and 2 medium slices of light white cheese .

Lunch:

Salad (mix of leaves, carrot, and cucumber, tomato and sesame seed) + 4 tbsp. (soup) cooked quinoa + 3 tbsp.

lentil (soup)   + 1 saucer of broccoli with olive oil and garlic + 1 medium portion of dogfish cooked with tomato and turmeric sauce.

Afternoon snack:

1 banana heated in the microwave with 1 tbsp. (dessert) of cocoa powder and chia.

To have lunch:

Muffin (2 beaten eggs, 3 teaspoons of oat bran, tuna, grated zucchini, salt, pepper, turmeric, olives – mix and bake in cupcake molds) + 1 saucer of vegetables (peppers, carrots, eggplant , tomato) roasted and seasoned with extra virgin olive oil and oregano.

Supper:

1 orange with pomace.

DAY 3 (40% CARBOHYDRATE)

Breakfast:

Overnight oat (1 tablespoon of vanilla whey protein with 1/2 pot of low-fat natural yogurt, 3 strawberries, 1 tablespoon of oat bran and 5 almonds – mix the ingredients the night before and leave in the refrigerator).

Morning snack:

1 cup. (Tea) of orange peel with ginger + 2 whole grain grissini with flaxseed.

Lunch:

Salad (mix of leaves, bean sprouts, red cabbage , edam-me (green soybeans) and sliced almonds with 3 tablespoons of vinaigrette (tomato, onion, olive oil and lemon)) + 2 medium slices of roasted pumpkin + 1 fillet (medium) of grilled lean meat.

Afternoon snack:

1 glass (200 ml) of low-fat natural yogurt mixed with 3 strawberries and 2 chopped Brazil nuts.

To have lunch:

1 saucer (tea) of sliced zucchini and tomato, roasted with 1 drizzle of olive oil, drops of lemon and orange and a little salt + 1 medium chicken fillet breaded with oats and roasted + sautéed spinach with cubes of white cheese.

Supper:

2 col. avocado (soup) with cocoa (1 drizzle of honey, if necessary).

DAY 4 (30% CARBOHYDRATE)

Breakfast:

Oat porridge – 1 ½ tbsp. (soup) of oat bran cooked in 1 glass (150 ml) of lactose-free milk (or vegetable milk), cinnamon and 1 tbsp. (tea) coconut sugar.

Morning snack:

Smoothie – 1 glass (200 ml) of low-fat natural yogurt mixed with 1 tbsp. (soup) vanilla whey protein, 1 tbsp. (soup) of oat bran and cinnamon powder.

Lunch:

Salad (mix of leaves, broccoli, peas , cherry tomatoes and chia seeds) + 1 medium slice of cooked sweet potato + 1 medium slice of roasted salmon afternoon snack + 5 rice crackers with a thin layer of peanut butter no sugar.

To have lunch:

2 wrap (cabbage leaf with lean ground beef, cottage cheese and grated carrot 1 medium piece of grilled peach palm).

Supper:

1 thin slice of melon (or 1 passion fruit).

DAY 5 (25% CARBOHYDRATE)

Breakfast:

2 scrambled eggs.

Morning snack:

Shake – 1/4 avocado shaken with coconut water , lemon and 1 drizzle of honey (optional).

Lunch:

Salad (mix of leaves with chia, sesame and sunflower seeds without the skin) + 1 medium fillet of roasted fish + 1 saucer of cooked chayote and seasoned with 1 drizzle of extra virgin olive oil and herbs.

Afternoon snack:

Shake – 1 glass (200 ml) of skimmed milk shaken with 1 tbsp. (soup) of vanilla whey protein and 2 chestnuts.

To have lunch:

1 tomato stuffed with roasted ricotta + 3 tons of zucchini spaghetti with Bolognese sauce (lean meat).

Supper:

1 col. pumpkin seed (soup).

CHAPTER 3

Low carb snacks to eat at work

Less refined carbohydrates, more real food: this is the proposal of many nutritionists for those who want to balance their diet and gain benefits such as weight loss – the so-called low carb diet.

This is because consuming excess carbohydrates promotes anxiety, depression and degenerative diseases, as their components inflame tissues and alter brain function.

For this reason, they are not the first option in the diet of those who spend all day at the office, sitting for more than eight hours. At these times, it's worth opting for low carb snacks.

If you are one of these people, stay calm. The solution to staying healthy is to reduce this food group from your menu (little by little) and eat low carb snacks to resist temptation.

When your stomach starts growling and you don't have any low carb snacks on hand, you know your only option is to head straight to the bakery. Store the healthy and smart options below in your drawer or desk:

Dry fruits

Any time of day is perfect to enjoy these delicacies, as they are high in protein, healthy fats and fiber. This combination of nutrients improves concentration, provides satiety and invigorates the body, making it one of the best snacks for work. It is worth consuming 30 to 50 grams per day to take advantage of its properties.

Strawberries with cottage cheese

Strawberries are an ideal food for the office due to their practicality to transport and the low amount of carbohydrates they contain (1 cup is equivalent to 11 g of carbohydrates) . Therefore, do not hesitate to include half a cup of this fruit in your daily life, combined with a serving of cottage cheese . This dairy product offers vitamins and minerals that control weight, stimulate intestinal health and activate brain function.

Apple with peanut butter

The combination of these two ingredients creates a delicious, slimming and energetic snack, as apples are rich in fiber and water, and peanut butter is rich in essential fatty acids. To make the most of its benefits, choose the version of the cream without added sugar.

Carrot and cucumber strips

Don't have much time to prepare a snack that makes you feel satisfied and helps your health? We have good news, carrots and cucumbers cut into strips are an excellent option. Firstly, because they combat constipation and fluid retention caused by stress at work, in addition to invigorating the mind, thanks to the minerals they contain.

Green smoothies

If you spend all day sitting at the office, you should definitely opt for a green smoothie. In addition to being refreshing and revitalizing, it improves digestion when there is little body movement. How to prepare them? Ideally, process a handful of green leaves, a piece of ginger, a portion of kiwi or apple to sweeten and water.

CHAPTER 4

Diet Mistakes You Make at Work

Snacks in the meeting room, birthday parties, coffee: there are many temptations that hinder the success of your diet at work.

But these are not the only reasons – nor the main ones – that are preventing you from following a healthier diet. Apparently innocent routine habits are the main diet mistakes and the most frequent weight loss saboteurs.

Check out five mistakes that are making results difficult on the scale – and find out how to avoid them.

Skipping breakfast to get to the office early

Of course, arriving early and being able to resolve pending issues while the phone doesn't ring and the email box doesn't fill up guarantees productivity. However, starting to work without fuel for your body makes you look for calories wherever you can find them. That famous stuffed cheese bread, for example. It's worth waking up a few minutes earlier to have enough time for a healthy breakfast at home. A combination of protein, complex carbohydrates and healthy fats is a good option. Think scrambled eggs with vegetables and whole-grain toast, or oatmeal with 2% milk, a tablespoon of nuts, and some fruit. If you're in a rush, pack a morning lunch to go with a low- sugar granola bar, two scrambled eggs, or fruit.

Accept everything colleagues offer

A little piece of chocolate here, a nut there, a bite of savory. This may all seem harmless. But the addition of calories from "snacking" on other people's sweets and snacks can result, over a period of two months, in a gain of one kilogram of body weight. Pay attention to why you are making these diet mistakes. You are hungry? Is it for social interaction? Just a habit?

Eat lunch at the table in front of the computer

This is a famous and frequent habit that is among diet mistakes. Because even if you're eating grilled chicken and salad, staring at your computer screen while eating lunch means you're not paying attention to how much food

you're consuming. It is no coincidence that mindful eating
, which advocates "eating consciously and paying attention
to the act of eating", is increasingly widespread. As
difficult as it may seem, do your best to step away from
your desk. For those times when you really can't get away,
halve your lunch to keep your portion in check, then save
the rest for a mid-afternoon snack when you have time for
a screen-free break.

Letting stress overwhelm you

Got nervous and attacked a cookie jar? This happens
because stress causes the body to release the hormone
cortical. In turn, blood sugar levels rise and fall, triggering
cravings for sugary, high-carb foods.

Remember that stress-related cravings are emotional – not
a sign that you're hungry. Instead of a cookie, what you
need is a calming tool. Take a deep breath; watch a funny
video on your phone, or text a friend.

Don't bring snacks from home

When your stomach starts growling and you don't have a
healthy snack on hand, your only option is to head straight
to the bakery. Store healthy and smart options in your
drawer or desk, such as unsweetened yogurt, mixed nuts

and fruits. But be aware of one catch: keeping these snacks nearby can make it easier to eat mindlessly throughout the day – and load up on extra calories that your body doesn't need. Portioning food prevents mistakes in the diet that many eat, as does limiting oneself to two snacks a day – one mid-morning and one in the afternoon, for example.

CHAPTER 5

Cheap weight loss menu: Healthy cheap diet

It's no secret that what you put on your plate plays a central role in weight loss. However, many people give up on starting the diet because they think about the costs they will incur. Well, the idea that you spend a lot to follow a healthier lifestyle soon appears. However, you don't have to spend a fortune to maintain a quality diet. In other words, it is possible to create a menu to lose weight cheaply. In other words, a cheap diet.

It is possible to lose weight with simple meal suggestions and affordable foods in your diet. This way, you won't need to buy anything special or invest in a dozen light or diet products.

Therefore, create a light menu and plan throughout the week to consume what you prepare at home. Furthermore, it is healthier and much cheaper than eating on the street.

Finally, check out our menu suggestions to lose weight on the cheap.

Cheap weight loss menu: Cheap diet

Rice and beans in the diet

The classic Brazilian combination is a great option to include in a simple and inexpensive diet. Well, these two foods form a nutritious and protein combination. Furthermore, it provides a cheap diet. But, if you can invest in brown rice, the benefits are even better.

Lean proteins for a cheap diet

- Lizard

- Muscle

- Liver

- Chicken fillet

- Egg

- Tilapia fillet

- Sardine

Cheap Diet: Cheap Whole Carbs

- Sweet potato

- Yam

- Cassava

- Brown rice

- Whole grain bread

- Oat

- Finally, whole wheat pasta

Good fats

- Chestnut and walnuts

- Extra virgin olive oil

- Avocado

- Linseed

- Wheezing

- Finally, olives

Cheap vegetables to include in your diet

- Pumpkin

- Tomato

- Beet

- Carrot

- Cucumber

- Chayote

- Lettuce

- Escarole

- Chard

- Additionally, arugula

- Fresh herbs

- Banana

- Litter

- Orange

- Pineapple

- Additionally, papaya

- Finally, melon

Cheap weight loss menu: Seasonings for a cheap diet

But, in addition to making food tastier, everyday spices such as pepper, cinnamon , ginger and mustard seed are considered thermogenic foods . Because, they "force" the body to spend more energy during digestion. In other words, they promote fat burning.

CHAPTER 6

8 thermogenic foods that are allies of the low carb diet

Thermogenic foods can be great allies of the low carb diet , as they require the body to burn more calories to digest them.

Basically, they work by increasing the body's temperature. Thus, causing the metabolism to be faster and fat burning to be much greater.

So, check out eight thermogenic foods that are part of a low carb menu:

Thermogenic foods that is friendly to the low carb diet

Cinnamon

This spice also prolongs satiety and reduces the desire to eat sweets. Cinnamon raises body temperature and regulates the release of insulin from the pancreas.

Ginger

Ginger stimulates the production of substances such as dopamine, which are responsible for promoting increased fat burning. Likewise, it reduces the absorption of ingested fat.

Red fruits

Fruits such as blackberries, strawberries and raspberries are rich in vitamin C, which is a natural antioxidant, and fiber, which prolongs the feeling of satiety and is essential for the intestinal tract. They also have a low sugar and calorie content.

Green Tea

Green tea contains substances such as caffeine and epigallocatechins that stimulate the use of fat stores as a source of energy, increasing the metabolic rate.

Red pepper

Stimulant, the seasoning increases salivation, stimulates gastric secretion and intestinal motility. Thus, some studies show a reduction in food intake and an increase in energy expenditure after meals containing pepper.

Chard

In addition to being low carb, the vegetable is rich in antioxidants that fight cell aging, preventing diseases such as cancer. Furthermore, thanks to the syringic acid present in the leaf, chard helps control blood sugar.

Asparagus

Low in calories, it deserves to be highlighted in weight loss plans, as it is rich in vitamins and fiber and helps to satisfy hunger. It also has a diuretic action, combating swelling and free radicals, which cause damage to the body.

Cabbage

Very healthy, kale is a famous leaf in the preparation of weight loss juices thanks to its low calorie content around 27 calories per 100g. It is also rich in fiber, which makes you feel full.

CHAPTER 7

Thermogenic juices that help you lose weight
Anyone trying to lose weight may have already opted for detox juices to help with the process. Lesser known, thermogenic juices are also healthy and help with weight loss.

First of all, do you know what thermogenic foods are? Thermogenic foods can be great allies in your diet as they require the body to burn more calories to digest them.

Basically, thermogenic juices work by increasing the body's temperature. Thus, causing the metabolism to be faster and fat burning to be much greater.

See thermogenic juice ideas

Watermelon juice with cinnamon

Watermelon is 92% water. Combined with water, the magnesium and potassium present in the fruit help with the discomfort caused by swelling. On hotter days, when the body tends to accumulate more fluids, the tip is to enjoy the fruit (a 100g portion has 31 kcal), whether in pieces or in the form of juice.

On the other hand, cinnamon stimulates digestion and even reduces "bad cholesterol" levels in the blood. Furthermore, it is even considered thermogenic. In other words, it is among the foods that "force" the body to spend more energy during digestion and, thus, promote weight loss.

Pineapple juice with ginger

Well known for being digestive and for its diuretic action, pineapple helps eliminate toxins. Furthermore, it is a natural antioxidant, that is, it contributes to the fight against premature aging in cell renewal.

Ginger is a natural thermogenic. It can also facilitate digestion and alleviate the discomfort of heartburn and abdominal bloating. Food is extremely accessible – it can be found at fairs, emporiums and supermarkets. However, to make juice with ginger and reap its benefits, prefer the pure root: just a small piece is enough to make the infusion.

Red fruit juice among thermogenic juices

Fruits such as blackberries, strawberries and raspberries are rich in vitamin C, which is a natural antioxidant, and fiber, which prolongs the feeling of satiety and is essential for the intestinal tract. Furthermore, they are low in sugar and calories.

Thermogenic juices: avocado with green tea

For those planning a diet , the good news is that avocados are rich in fatty acids. But especially omegas 6, 7 and 9. By balancing the body, they help with fat loss. Components such as fiber, phytosterols and oleic acid increase the feeling of satiety, reduce binge eating and reduce the accumulation of fat in the abdominal region.

Meanwhile, green tea has an important antioxidant function, which contributes to the prevention of cardiovascular diseases, diabetes and cancer, for example. Among other benefits, green tea speeds up metabolism, making you burn fat faster and thus lose weight.

Furthermore, the catechins in its composition interact with leptin receptors, a hormone related to the body's feeling of satiety, preventing you from eating more than your body needs.

CHAPTER 8

Thermogenic tea helps you lose and maintain weight.

Teas are true allies for those who are going through a weight loss process. This is because the drink helps the body to debloat and get rid of fluid retention. But did you know that some strategies can enhance the power of drinks? For example, preparing a thermogenic tea, that is, with ingredients that help the body burn even more calories. At this time, it's worth using creativity and varying the types of foods, such as ginger, cinnamon and even pepper. Check out some tips!

Thermogenic tea: benefits

Accelerating metabolism is the main objective of thermogenic tea. This occurs because the drink contains substances that require more effort than usual to be digested. Thus, the body uses more energy and makes the metabolism work harder, increasing calorie burning even at rest.

In other words, when combined with a balanced diet and frequent physical exercise, thermogenic teas are capable of accelerating the calorie burning process. Check out some options:

Ginger

Speeds up metabolism and helps with healthy weight loss. It is antioxidant, anti-inflammatory, tonic and expectorant. Furthermore, it aids digestion. People with heart problems should be careful with excessive use, as it accelerates the heart rate. Patients with hyperthyroidism should also be careful. See how to prepare.

Green Tea

Green tea stimulates energy expenditure and helps with fat loss. Furthermore, it helps the metabolism to function properly. However, excessive consumption can be harmful to the body. As it contains caffeine, use in large quantities can cause insomnia, in addition to leading to gastritis, as it increases gastric flow. Pregnant women, people with hyperthyroidism and patients with hypertension, glaucoma and gastric problems should avoid it. Check out a recipe.

Cinnamon

Cinnamon tea speeds up metabolism, reduces appetite, has anti-inflammatory and antibacterial effects, and improves blood circulation. However, excessive consumption can cause allergic skin problems and cause insomnia. Pregnant women cannot consume it.

Thermogenic tea: hibiscus tea

Hibiscus is a medicinal plant with thermogenic properties capable of accelerating calorie burning. The plant also has a diuretic effect, which contributes to reducing fluid retention, as well as helping to regulate cholesterol and prevent cell aging. It is not recommended for pregnant and lactating women.

Clove

Clove is a powerful thermogenic, capable of accelerating metabolism and enhancing weight loss. Furthermore, it has properties that help with digestion, favoring the proper functioning of the intestine. Pregnant women, those who are breastfeeding and children under six years of age should avoid drinking the drink. Understand better.

Black pepper

Pepper tea helps with weight loss, as the ingredient has thermogenic properties that help accelerate metabolism.

After all, does thermogenic tea help you lose weight?

Thermogenic teas accelerate metabolism and enhance fat burning. However, just drinking the tea does not cause weight loss. The benefits of thermogenic teas can only be achieved as long as consumption of the drink is associated with a healthy eating routine and regular physical exercise. Also, talk to a healthcare professional before adding the drink to your menu.

CHAPTER 9

Thermogenic recipes to include in your diet

Ingredients: Thermogenic Seasoning

0.5 teaspoons of Master foods Calabria pepper

0.5 teaspoons of Ginger powder

5.0 grams of raw Garlic

This recipe may contain brand suggestions for reference only when calculating nutritional information. Feel free to choose the product from the supplier or manufacturer you prefer.

How to make thermogenic seasoning

Mix all ingredients in a seasoning container, preferably glass.

Thermogenic Seasoning Nutritional Information

Grams Per Serving: 9 g

- Calories 8.05 kcal

- Carbohydrates1.73g

- Proteins0.40 g

- Total fat0.03 g

- Gord. Saturated0.01 g

- Gord. trans0.00 g

- Fibers0.28g

- Sodium0.64m

Thermogenic cappuccino recipe

There's never a bad time for a cup of coffee, much less for a delicious cappuccino. What if it's a version that, in addition to being tasty, contributed to weight loss? Next, check out a recipe for thermogenic cappuccino!

The drink, which has up to 88 calories per serving, can be a great addition to your diet . This is because the preparation method uses thermogenic nutrients basically, these foods act by increasing the body's temperature, causing the metabolism to accelerate and fat burning to be greater. **Find out how to prepare:**

Thermogenic cappuccino recipe

Ingredients:

- 1 teaspoon of sugar - free soluble coffee powder;

- 1 teaspoon of honey or sweetener;

- 1 tablespoon (dessert) of hot water;

- 1 cup (tea) of skimmed milk;

- 1 teaspoon of cocoa powder;

- Cinnamon powder to taste.

Method of preparation:

First, mix the coffee, honey and hot water until it forms foam. Then, heat the milk and mix it with the cocoa and cinnamon. Finally, just add it to the coffee and serve it hot!

Thermogenic Broth

Ingredients of: **Thermogenic Broth** (Clear)

1.0 medium unit of cooked Carrot

1.0 medium unit of cooked beetroot

1.0 medium unit of raw yellow pepper

1.0 medium unit of cooked sweet potato

Black pepper powder to taste

Extra virgin olive oil to taste

1.0 tablespoon of garlic powdeR

How to make Thermogenic Broth

In 500 ml of water cook the sweet potato, carrot and beetroot. After cooking for 10 minutes, set aside the vegetables and sauté in olive oil with garlic and chopped pepper. In a blender or processor, add the water used to prepare the vegetables, the same sautéed vegetables and black pepper, blending until a paste with the texture of broth is formed.

Thermogenic Broth Nutritional Information

Grams per Serving: 298 g

- Calories160.60 kcal

- Carbohydrates37.62 g

- Proteins2.55 g

- Total fat0.43g

- Gord. Saturated0.00 g

- Gord. trans0.00 g

- Fibers6.50 g

- Sodium23.02mg

Summer thermogenic shot

Ingredients of: **Summer Thermogenic** Shot (Clear)

0.5 teaspoons of cinnamon powder

1.0 teaspoon (tea) Ginger powder

0.5 teaspoons of saffron powder

Red or cayenne pepper to taste

50.0 milliliters of water

0.5 units of lemon juice

How to do a summer thermogenic shot

In a glass, mix the ingredients and drink immediately.

Summer Thermogenic Shot Nutritional Information

Grams Per Serving: 80 g

- Calories25.11 kcal

- Carbohydrates5.72g

- Proteins0.53g

- Total fat0.42 g

- Gord. Saturated0.02 g

- Gord. trans0.00 g

- Fibers0.54 g

- Sodium2.28 mg

Thermogenic Avocado Cream

Ingredients: Thermogenic Avocado Cream (Clear)

1.0 average unit of Avocado

1.0 milliliter of unsweetened lemon juice

1.0 pot of Nestlé traditional light Greek yogurt

100.0 grams of Native organic demerara sugar

1.0 tablespoon Fit União refined sugar

10.0 grams of Ginger

How to make thermogenic avocado cream

Place all the ingredients except the dried fruits, carob and sweetener in a blender and blend well until smooth. Consume next.

Nutritional Information for Thermogenic Avocado Cream

Grams Per Serving: 641 g

- Calories938.00 kcal

- Carbohydrates146.93g

- Proteins10.34g

- Total fat53.87g

- Gord. Saturated11.01g

- Gord. trans0.00 g

- Fibers27.29g

- Sodium61.31 mg

CHAPTER 10

Mindful Eating: The method that teaches you how to eat consciously

Try to eat consciously, understanding the type of food you are eating and the taste, in order to extract the maximum benefit. This is what mindful eating preaches, an ancient technique widely used in behavioral nutrition and which proposes awareness of signs and responses to the act of nourishment, maintaining curiosity in seeking to perceive sensations.

Contrary to traditional diets , in which food is controlled or imposed, the mindful eating method helps to connect mind and body and, thus, build a healthier relationship with food.

What is mindful eating?

Mindful eating, in a literal translation, means eating with full attention. "The technique poses a challenge to modern society, without time, to redirect, raise awareness and have full lucidity when eating", says Dr. Fernanda Vasconcelos, nutritionist at Hospital Santa Cruz, in São Paulo.

According to the expert, to eat consciously you need to understand the sensations involved in the entire process of eating, both physically and emotionally. From hunger, choosing food, preparing the menu and feeling full when we are satisfied after finishing the meal.

Therefore, very simple guidelines can have a great effect on the results. "Start meals with a salad, have no food on the table (ready-made dish), and eat consciously and slowly. Because the rhythm of the meal is important to recognize the satiety response — and this takes on average 20 minutes after the start of the meal", explains Michael Zanchet, a clinical psychologist specializing in health behaviors, stress and anxiety .

"Every time you think about the possibility of eating some food, therefore, reflect and ask yourself: 'How long ago did I eat my last meal?'. If it was less than three hours ago, ask yourself again: 'What are you hungry for?', adds the specialist. "If it lasts three hours or more, it is probably a nutritional need, but if the period is shorter, it could be anxiety, sadness or even thirst."

Mindful eating x weight loss

According to mindful eating, neither extreme is "right" when it comes to eating. If the relationship with food is not good, it becomes an obsession, increasing dissatisfaction and insecurity, which leads to bad choices at the table, in a vicious circle.

Therefore, although it is not a diet (the technique does not work with restrictions, eating plans, calorie counting or prohibited foods), this concept can help with weight control. "The difference is that this method seeks to provide a new relationship with food. Changing the habit of eating disorganized and seeking to carry this solidified habit into life", guarantees the psychologist.

"So, rejecting the diet mentality is the first step in intuitive eating, seeking a healthier relationship with food. Therefore, they are practices that are very different from the usual prescriptions of a diet and seek to reconnect with the internal signs of dietary regulation", says the doctor.

Food philosophy also seeks to teach how to distinguish physical hunger amidst the release of different simultaneous sensations produced in everyday life . "Many people eat in an attempt to fill another void, which is not hunger, but rather boredom, sadness, anxiety or stress. This discernment is fundamental", says the nutritionist. "Reading, listening to music, watching television, using your cell phone or tablet tends to defocus our attention from food and, furthermore, predispose us to overeating. This is very harmful, and goes against the process of full attention and awareness during meals", she adds.

The benefits of mindful eating

Anxiety, binge eating, mood disorders, depression , post-traumatic stress, chronic pain, cancer, substance abuse, among many other clinical conditions. All of them can be better managed through the practice of mindful eating.

Therefore, for those who adopt this style of eating, a series of benefits have already been noticed. Reduction in risk factors for eating disorders, reduction in compulsions related to food, less internalization of thin ideals, association with pleasure in eating, less dieting and less anxiety about eating.

"The method also allows for awareness of oneself, one's own actions, with recovery of self-control and self-confidence, giving less chance to unwanted, thoughtless behaviors, exaggerations and compulsions. Thus, all of this reflects in the reduction of BMI (body mass index), with an improvement in the metabolic profile and psychological health", guarantees the specialist.

Tips for practicing mindful eating

Before eating

First, carefully prepare your own food, paying attention to every detail. This is all part of the eating process. Thus, mindful eating is an invitation to lucidity of all these sensations.

Sit down to eat instead of standing in front of the refrigerator, following "pinching" patterns, which hinder awareness of the meal in terms of both quality and quantity. Next, pay attention to the intensity of your hunger this is how your body tells you that your energy levels are getting low and that it will soon be time to replenish your fuel.

Generally, hunger is caused by biological factors. But it can also be triggered by feelings (anxiety, sadness and anger, for example). In this case, it is called emotional hunger.

Knowing how to differentiate between physiological and emotional hunger, as well as identifying its size, is very important to find out if you really need to eat at that moment (and if so, how large a portion you should put on your plate). This avoids exaggeration.

Finally, dedicate yourself absolutely to each and every meal, avoiding sharing your attention with other activities or distractions, such as electronic devices. Look at the dish and use your senses: before taking the first bite, feel the aromas, texture and even the sound of it.

During the meal

Enjoy every bite: try to chew as much as possible and breathe calmly. Therefore, between bites, place your fork on the table and only pick it up again when you have finished swallowing. After the first few minutes, reduce the amount of food you put in your mouth.

Observe how the food behaves inside the oral cavity: does it melt, bubble or is it resistant? Also, notice what you are feeling at the moment. Food diaries can help people become more aware and visualize what they are eating. Not everyone has this availability and organization to do it, but those who do can benefit from the habit.

Exaggerated? See what to do

No guilt and much less punishments and restrictions! So, know that it's all part of a process, and try again at the next meal.

Mindful eating tips for beginners

If you have never practiced mindful eating and had no idea what it was until you read our content, check out some tips to start the technique:

- Regular training: it doesn't matter if it's just a few minutes a day consistency will make all the difference in being able to incorporate the practice into your meals;

- Meditate: set aside five minutes at the end of the day to work on mindfulness (there are great apps that help you with this);

- Stay away from devices: try to eat in a place without cell phones, TVs, tablets or any electronic device that could disturb the moment;

- Start slowly: first, choose just one meal a day to train mindfulness;

- Notice everything: look at the colors on your plate, smell the food, notice the quantities chosen and feel the flavor and texture of the prepared recipes.

<u>Detox: Body and mind</u>

Difficulty meditating? 4 solutions to common problems when practicing

When we talk about the main self-care trends, meditation is definitely on the list. And for good reason: it has been proven to help in different areas of life from relieving anxiety to even improving your sex life. However, if you have tried (and tried, and tried…) to do the act without success, don't feel alone. See tips on how to overcome the main challenges faced by those who have difficulty meditating:

Difficulty meditating

I can't clear my mind

Legs crossed, eyes closed, body relaxed — you're ready for a meditation session. However, there's just one problem: you can't stop thinking about all the items on your to-do list, that fight you just had with your sister, or what you're making for dinner. Sound familiar? No matter how hard we try, sometimes it is absolutely impossible to completely empty our mind.

If you are having difficulty staying focused , we suggest trying mindfulness meditation. Therefore, with this type of meditation, the objective is not to completely clear the mind of all thoughts; rather, it is being fully aware of your thoughts and surroundings in the present moment. So if your mind wanders, just notice that your mind is wandering and be aware of it so you can get back to focusing.

Additionally, a guided meditation can help improve your concentration there are several free apps that offer this service!

Difficulty meditating: I feel restless

Many people feel agitated when they try to meditate. In order to be more comfortable and at peace with our lives, we need to learn to deal with this restlessness in a different way and learn to resolve it. Try different types of meditation . Your restlessness may be suited to a walking meditation, in which you focus on staying mentally present while moving your body.

I have no time

Having time for this self-care practice can be very good for your body and mind. This is because studies have shown that mediation can increase immunity. But there's more: it is capable of sharpening memory, relieving chronic pain, reducing depression and anxiety and improving sleep.

Furthermore, meditation does not have to last for hours and hours. You can start with just three minutes a day, for example.

Difficulty meditating: Causes (a lot of) sleep

An alternative is to practice meditation right before bedtime. This way, the body will feel ready to rest. Also, if you are prone to drowsiness but are determined to stay awake for an entire session, choose a time of day when you tend to feel least tired.

CHAPTER 11

Meditation: what it is, benefits, what it is for and how to do it

More than closing your eyes and remaining silent, meditation is a set of concentration techniques that aim to achieve mental and emotional plenitude. The benefits of this ancient practice for health and well-being are already more than proven. Its origin is not known for sure, but it is part of the tradition of many peoples and cultures, such as Indian and Japanese.

Importance of meditation

Meditation helps reduce stress in our lives by putting the body in a relaxed state. Every time we sit, we are literally inviting our cells to release stress reactions that we have built up over time, leaving us clearer, brighter, balanced and adaptable.

Through meditation, we can find levels of happiness, which become more and more accessible the more we practice. Additionally, meditation reduces blood pressure , improves sleep , and increases the overall sense of contentment and roundedness.

Main types of meditation

Despite presenting different proposals, all meditations have the objective of leading you to delve into yourself for self-knowledge. In other words, it is this experience that will free the individual from anxiety and other disorders that are so common in our modern society.

Mindfulness

It is the best known modality in the Western world. In this way, it was disconnected from religious beliefs and is based on techniques approved by science. Thus, Mindfulness meditation focuses on concentration exercises and attention to physical sensation and breathing. In other words, it eliminates the need to chant mantras. "Just have any free moment of the day to enjoy the benefits. Furthermore, choosing a quiet place is essential to help you pay attention to what is happening to your body", advises Maria Helena Garcia, coach and Mindfulness meditation teacher.

But, to feel the effects of the practice, the coach suggests eight weeks of daily exercises (of course, it is desirable that you continue meditating after this period). "So, five minutes to start. When you get used to it, increase it little by little, until you reach 20 minutes", says the specialist.

Transcendental meditation

Transcendental meditation is another way to experience states of tranquility, relaxation, and mindfulness. Based on the teachings of master Maharishi Mahesh Yogi, the technique also seeks concentration and mind control. In this way, the person practically effortlessly reaches the fourth state of consciousness, where we are not sleeping, dreaming or awake, we are relaxed. According to the Transcendental Meditation website, this is the experience of transcendence, which creates the ideal condition to activate the innate power that the body has to restore itself.

In addition to the benefits mentioned above, TM also promises to help reduce other problems such as panic syndrome, risk of stroke, hypertension and heart attack, because it acts directly on the nervous system. But, to reach this statement, 600 practical studies were carried out monitoring the effect of the technique on volunteers.

Zazen

Za means to sit; Zen represents a state of deep and subtle meditation. Just like other types of meditation, it is necessary to remain seated, inviting the practitioner to pay attention to their physical posture from the beginning of the process. In other words, the teacher leads the practitioner into a narrative for introspection and awareness by inhaling and releasing air.

1.   Choose a quiet place where you will not be interrupted. Dress comfortably;

2.   To start, sit with your legs crossed on the zafu – a round cushion specifically for this meditation – with your knees resting on the floor;

3.   Keep your eyes half-open and your vision at a 45-degree angle. It is also important to maintain the right posture, with a straight spine, elongated neck and ears towards the shoulders; this allows the diaphragm to open and facilitates the passage of vital energy;

4.   Then do the cosmic mudra. Place the back of the fingers of your left hand over the fingers of your right hand and the tips of your thumbs lightly touching each other;

5.   Inhale and exhale deeply, then open your mouth to exhale smoothly and slowly. Exhale all the air from your lungs. After three deep breaths, close your mouth and breathe naturally through your nostrils;

6.   When you finish zazen, place your hands on your thighs with your palms facing up. If you need to, shake your body a few times and inhale deeply. Uncross your legs and start moving slowly again.

Vipassana meditation

It is one of the oldest meditation techniques, originating from India 2,500 years ago. Vipassana means "seeing things as they really are". This type of meditation is taught in immersive courses that last 10 days. During this period, basic concepts of the method and their practice are learned.

To be successful in obtaining the benefits, you must be committed to meditation, following some codes of discipline transmitted during the course, such as abstaining from sex, lying and toxic substances (narcotics and alcohol, for example). This temporary abdication helps to calm the mind for the exercise of self-observation. Such steps will lead to the development of mastery of the mind, in order to focus attention on the way one breathes , sits, among other physical and mental sensations.

Candle meditation

Candle meditation – also called Trataka – consists of firmly fixing your gaze on a candle without blinking, until you tear up. Trataka provides deep cleaning of the eyes and tears serve as a mechanism for eliminating toxins from our body.

Therefore, through candle meditation, it is possible to rest your vision and tone your eye muscles. Consequently, it contributes to the prevention and treatment of various vision problems.

One of the biggest benefits of candle meditation is increasing focus and concentration, eliminating distractions and negative thoughts. This is because with the light and heat of the candle, it becomes easier to keep your attention just on it.

Check out the step-by-step guide on how to do this type of meditation:

1.   Light a candle, you can choose any type;

2.   Don't forget to dim the light in the room so that the candle flame stands out;

3.   Then, place the candle on a table, about 50 centimeters away and sit on a chair in front of it;

4.   Remain seated with your back straight and take slow, deep breaths. This way, the aim is to relax;

5.   Therefore, your attention should only be focused on the candle flame;

6.   Get rid of any thoughts that may distract your mind. So if this happens, bring your mind back to the candle;

7.   Finally, blink after seeing the tears flow.

Compassion meditation

Compassion meditation involves silently repeating a few phrases that move from judgment to care, from isolation to connection, and from indifference to understanding. When practicing it, the pro-social areas of the brain are activated. These areas of the brain are also stimulated when you are with friends or family.

Learn how to perform compassion meditation:

1.	You can start with a 20-minute session and gradually increase the time until you are meditating for half an hour a day;

2.	First, find an object to focus on freely. Observe the object and leave your attention only to that. This will help create a sense of awareness of what is happening to your mind and at the same time the mind slows down;

3.	Now, think about a loved one. When you are focused within, shift your attention to a loved one who makes you happy. When we see our loved ones happy and smiling it brings us a smile too;

4.	Then, imagine good vibrations for the person you love, removing any type of anxiety or suffering that they may be going through.

5.	Bring your intentions inward, focus on the object, and finish by focusing on your breath. You always begin and end compassion meditation with a sense of mindfulness.

6.	Although a normal meditation may take a few minutes, it is recommended to carry this practice with you throughout the day. At any moment, worry about the outside world starts to overwhelm you, so it's important to stay focused on practice.

Body Scan Meditation

Body scanning meditation, a practice that involves consciously scanning your body for sensations of pain, tension, and other unusual things. Thus, the technique is a type of meditation in which you must pay attention to each limb, from head to toe. See step by step how to do it:

1.   Lie down or sit in a position that allows you to stretch your limbs easily. Then, close your eyes and start focusing on your breathing;

2.   Start wherever you want, whether it's your hands, feet or top of your head. Focus on that location while continuing to breathe slowly and deeply;

3.   Soon after, open your awareness to sensations of pain, tension, discomfort or anything out of the ordinary. Spend 20 seconds to 1 minute observing these sensations;

4.   If you begin to feel pain and discomfort, acknowledge and sit with the emotions these sensations bring up. For example, if you feel frustrated and angry, don't judge yourself for those emotions;

5.   Continue breathing, imagining the pain and tension decreasing with each breath;

6.   In this way, release your mental awareness in that specific part of your body and redirect it to your next area of focus;

7.   As you continue to scan your body, notice when your thoughts begin to drift. This will probably happen more than once, so don't worry;

8.   After you finish scanning parts of your body, let your awareness move through your body. Visualize this as liquid filling a mold. Continue breathing in and out slowly as you sit with this awareness of your whole body for a few seconds;

9.   Slowly release your focus and turn your attention to your surroundings.

Mindful eating: meditation while eating

Mindful eating basically consists of eating consciously. In other words, try to eat more consciously, noticing the type of food you are eating, the taste, the texture and the smell. Find out how to practice it:

1.   Dedicate yourself completely to each and every meal, avoiding sharing your attention with other activities or distractions — electronic devices, for example;

2.   Sit down to eat instead of standing in front of the refrigerator;

3.   Enjoy every bite: so, pay attention to the smell, temperature and texture of the food;

4.   Food diaries can help people have greater awareness and visualization of what they are eating;

5.   Finally, carefully prepare your own food, paying attention to every detail.

CHAPTER 12

Benefits of meditation

Focus on the "here and now"

"In an immediate society, meditating is an act of slowing down and respecting your own time, focusing your attention on the present moment", explains the coach. According to the expert, it is normal to cling to facts from the past, with thoughts such as 'If I had acted like that...', 'It could have been different if I had said that...', and future projections, such as thinking about the supermarket list when waking up or making vacation plans.

"The daily exercise of meditation helps us look at where we are now. How am I feeling? What am I eating? The perception of presence becomes more effective, and the individual begins to have more self-knowledge and attention to what really matters", says Maria Helena.

Anxiety relief

Anxiety is a result of thoughts focused on the future. It comes from uncertainties and facts that, in most cases, are not under our control. When you pay more attention to what you are thinking and doing, anxiety about the future decreases. The reason? We realize that it is not worth being nervous or anxious about situations that are independent of our will. When you meditate, you become more aware of what causes you frustration, imbalance, and discomfort, and you learn to direct these emotions.

According to research by the Brain Institute of Hospital Israelita Albert Einstein, eight weeks of practicing relaxing activities, in addition to breathing, attention and positive psychology reduced symptoms of stress by 35.3%, 27.84% of sadness and worry and 14% of emotions (fear and irritation, for example).

Reduces stress

"In addition to getting out of 'autopilot', a few minutes of introspection, in silence and breathing consciously are capable of relieving moments of tension and nervousness inherent to everyday life", explains the Mindfulness instructor.

Meditation helps in curing depression

Meditation can help reverse depression symptoms. "Regular practice can alter brain activity and neuron activity, breaking pessimistic thought patterns typical of depression ," he explains. However, you need to seek professional help before betting all your money on just one meditative technique.

Meditation FAQs

1) What is the easiest way to start making meditation part of your routine?

An alternative is to set the alarm clock to go off 20 minutes earlier. Brush your teeth and sit wherever you prefer couch, chair or floor. Get comfortable and let the show begin. At first, it will feel like you are being bombarded this is just your internal cleansing happening. Thoughts will be displayed in your consciousness. Therefore, observe and continue returning your attention to your breathing. It may take a few minutes, but the parade of thoughts will subside.

2) How often or for how long should beginners meditate?

Try it daily for 15 minutes for a week, and see how it goes. After all, a little meditation is better than none.

3) What is the best time of day to meditate?

There are no rules about when to meditate. Just define what time of day works best, taking into account your routine, including work, studies, children, among others. Therefore, try meditating in the morning, afternoon and **evening to reach a conclusion.**

How to start meditating

Step 1: **Set aside time**

Start by setting aside time in your day to practice meditation. It could be when you wake up, so you can start the day well; throughout the day, to de-stress the mind; or, at night, to ensure quality sleep .

Five minutes is enough for those just starting out — but the ideal is 15 to 20 minutes of full concentration. Over time, you will want to increase this period more and more. To remember, set your cell phone alarm clock.

Step 2: Choose a calm location

Whether in your bedroom, in your garden or even in your living room — the important thing is that the space is peaceful. Furthermore, turn off the TV and electronic devices in the room, put your cell phone on airplane

mode, and look for a quieter place, away from distractions.
If you can wear comfortable clothes and dim the light ,
the better;

Step 3: **Adopt a comfortable posture**

Most prefer the lotus posture — in which you sit, cross
your legs, maintain an upright posture and rest your hands
on your knees. But nothing stops you from practicing in
other positions, including lying down! So, prioritize the
way that makes you most comfortable.

Step 4: **Pay attention to your breathing**

Make sure you are breathing in and out correctly. In other
words, fill your lungs with air using your belly muscles,
and release it little by little during a slow and pleasant
exhalation.

Step 5: **Unclog**

Many people think they can't meditate because their mind
keeps wandering in thoughts. But "not thinking about
anything" requires many years of practice! So give it a try.
However, if you notice that you are "travelling", refocus.

CHAPTER 13

low-carb diet

A low-carb diet means you eat fewer carbohydrates and a higher proportion of fat. Even more important, you minimize your sugar and flour/starch intake. You can eat other delicious foods until you're full – and still lose weight.

A number of recent high-quality studies show that LCHF makes it easier to lose weight and control your blood sugar. And that's just the beginning.

The basic

Eat: meat, fish, eggs, vegetables that grow above ground and natural fats (such as butter)

Avoid: sugar and starchy foods (such as bread, pasta, rice and potatoes)

Eat when you are hungry, until you are satisfied. It's that simple. You don't need to count calories or weigh your food. And simply forget low-fat industrialized products.

Real food. Add some good fat (like butter)

There are solid scientific reasons why LCHF works. When you avoid sugar and starches, your blood sugar stabilizes and levels of insulin, the fat-storing hormone, drop. This increases your fat burning and makes you feel fuller.

Note for diabetics

Avoiding carbohydrates that increase your blood sugar levels reduces your need for medication to control it. Taking the same dose of pre-low-carb insulin when dieting can result in hypoglycemia (low blood sugar). You need to test your blood sugar frequently when starting the diet and adapt (reduce) your medication. This should ideally be done with the assistance of a doctor. If you are healthy or diabetic treated with some type of diet or just Metformin, there is no risk of hypoglycemia.

Nutritional advice

Eat whatever you want:

Meat: of any type, including beef, pork, game meat, chicken, etc. Feel free to eat the fat in meats as well as the skin of the chicken. If possible, choose to eat "organic" meat.

Fish and crustaceans: of all types. Fatty fish such as salmon, mackerel or herring are great.

Avoid breading

Eggs: in all forms. Boiled, fried, omelets, etc. Give preference to "organic" eggs

Natural sauces, with a lot of fat: using butter and cream when you cook can make your food tastier and make you feel fuller. Try béarnaise or hollandaise sauce, check the ingredients or make it yourself. Coconut and olive oils are also good options.

Vegetables that grow above ground: cauliflower, broccoli, cabbage, kale, Brussels sprouts. Asparagus, zucchini, eggplant, olives, spinach, mushrooms, cucumber, lettuce, abacte, pepper, tomatoes, etc.

Dairy products: always choose whole products, no skimmed products: butter, cream (40% fat), sour cream, Greek yogurt, yellow cheeses. Be cautious with milk and skimmed milk, as both contain a lot of lactose (milk sugar). Avoid flavored, sweetened and fat-free products.

Oilseeds: macadamias, hazelnuts, walnuts, Brazil nuts, cashew nuts, etc. Good to eat in front of the TV (**preferably in moderation**)

Fruits (strawberry, cherry, cherry, acerola, blackberry, and blueberry): to eat in moderation, if you do not adopt a super-restrictive diet or if you are not allergic. They are good with whipped cream.

Basic tip for beginners: maximum of 5 grams of carbohydrates (excluding fiber) per 100g of food.

Avoid if you can

Sugar: the worst of all. Soft drinks, sweets, juices, isotonic drinks, chocolates, cakes, bread, confectionery, snacks, ice cream, breakfast cereal. Preferably, avoid sweeteners too.

Starch: bread, pasta, rice, potatoes, porridge, musli and so on. "Whole products" are just less bad. Moderate amounts of roots and tubers may be ok (unless you choose to be "extremely low carb")

Margarine: industrial imitation of butter with artificially high omega-6 fat content. It has no health benefits.

Statistically, it is linked to asthma, allergies and other inflammatory diseases

Beer: it's liquid bread. Full of quickly absorbed carbohydrates, unfortunately.

Fruits: very sweet, involves a lot of sugar. Eat from time to time. Treat fruits as a form of "natural candy."

Sometimes

You decide when the time is right. Your weight loss may be slowed down a little.

Alcohol: dry wine (white or red), whiskey, cognac, vodka and sugar-free cocktails.

Dark chocolate: above 70% cocoa, preferably in small quantities.

Always drink: water, coffee (try with cream), tea

The theory behind LCHF

What were you designed to eat?

Humans evolved for millions of years as hunter-gatherers, without eating large amounts of carbohydrates. We ate the food available to us in nature by hunting, fishing, and collecting whatever edible items we could find. These foods did not include pure starch in the form of bread, pasta, rice or potatoes. We have been eating these foods for 5, 10 thousand years, since the development of agriculture. Only a limited adaptation of our genes happens in such a relatively short time.

With the Industrial Revolution 100-200 years ago, we built factories that could produce large quantities of sugar and white flour. Pure carbohydrates quickly digested. We barely had time to genetically adapt to such processed foods.

In the 1980s, the fear of fat captured the Western world. Low-fat products appeared everywhere. But if you eat less fat, you need to eat more carbohydrates to feel full. And it was at this moment in history that our disastrous obesity and diabetes epidemics began. As the most fat-scared country in the world, the USA was hit hardest and is now the most obese country on the planet.

Today, it is clear that the fear of real food with natural fat levels was a big mistake.

The problem with sugar and starch

All digestible carbohydrates are broken down into simple sugars in the intestines. The sugar is then absorbed into the blood, increasing the blood glucose level. This increases the production of insulin, our fat-storing hormone.

CHAPTER 14

Lack of food (especially carbohydrates) decreases insulin

Insulin is produced in the pancreas (illustrated on the right). In large amounts, insulin prevents fat burning and stores excess nutrients in fat cells. After some time (a few hours or less) this can result in a lack of nutrients in the blood, creating a feeling of hunger and an uncontrollable desire for something sweet. Usually at this point, people eat again. This starts the process all over again: a vicious cycle leading to weight gain.

On the other hand, a low carbohydrate intake gives you a lower, more stable blood glucose level and lower amounts of insulin. This increases the release of fat from your stores and increases burning – generally leading to fat loss, especially in the abdominal region, in obese individuals.

Weight loss without hunger

An LCHF diet makes it easier for the body to use its fat stores, as their release is no longer blocked by insulin levels. This may be one reason why eating fat gives you a longer-lasting feeling of fullness than carbohydrates. The fact has already been demonstrated in some studies: when people eat everything they want on a low carb diet, the amount of calories ingested typically decreases.

Therefore, counting or weighing the food is unnecessary. You can forget about calories and trust your feelings of hunger and satiety. Most people don't need to count or weigh their food any more than they need to count their exhales and inhales. If you don't believe it, try it for a few weeks and see for yourself.

Health as a bonus

No animal in nature needs the assistance of nutrition experts or calorie charts to eat. And yet, as long as they eat the food they evolved to eat, they remain at a normal weight and avoid cavities, diabetes and heart disease. Why would humans be an exception? Why would you be an exception?

In scientific studies, not only weight improves on a low carb diet – blood pressure, blood glucose and cholesterol indicators (HDL, triglycerides) also improve. A calm stomach and fewer cravings for sweet foods are also common experiences.

Initial side effects

If you stop eating sugar and starches abruptly (recommended), you may experience some side effects while your body adapts. For most people the effects tend to be mild and only last a few days. There are also ways to minimize them.

Common during the first week:

Headache

Fatigue

Dizziness

Palpitations

Irritability

Side effects quickly disappear as your body adapts and your fat burning increases. They can be minimized by drinking more fluids and temporarily increasing your salt intake. A good option is to drink broth every few hours. Or drink a few extra glasses of water and add more salt to your food.

The reason for this is that carbohydrate-rich foods increase water retention in your body. When you stop eating high-carb foods, you will lose excess water through your kidneys. This can result in dehydration and lack of salt for the first week, before the body adapts.

Some people prefer to decrease their carbohydrate intake slowly, over a few weeks, to minimize the effects. But the "Nike way" is probably the best choice for most people. Removing most of the sugar and starch usually results in losing a few pounds on the scale within a few days. The majority may be liquids, but they are very good for motivation.

How little (carbohydrate) to eat?

The fewer carbohydrates you eat, the more pronounced the effect will be on your weight and blood sugar. I recommend following nutritional directions as closely as you can. Once you're happy with your weight and health, you can gradually try eating more liberally (if you want).

The food revolution

Presentation by me at the 2011 Ancestral Health Symposium, summarizing the history and science behind the LCHF revolution

Tips and recipes

Breakfast suggestions

Eggs with bacon

Omelette

Leftovers from last night's dinner

Coffee with cream

Canned tuna with boiled eggs

Boiled eggs with mayonnaise or butter

Avocado, salmon and sour cream

Sandwich on flourless bread

A very thin piece of hard bread with plenty of butter, cheese, ham , etc.

Cheese with butter

Boiled eggs mashed with butter, chopped chives, salt and pepper

A piece of brie cheese with ham or salami

Full-fat yogurt with nuts and seeds (and perhaps berries)

Lunch and dinner

Dishes with meat, fish or chicken with vegetables and a high-fat sauce. There are many alternatives to mashed potatoes, such as cauliflower mash.

Stews, soups or casseroles with low carb ingredients.

You can use most recipes in books if you avoid high-carb ingredients. It's a good idea to add fat (butter, cream) to the recipe.

Drink water with your meal or (occasionally) a glass of wine.

Snacks

When you eat a low-carb diet with more fat and a little more protein, you probably won't need to eat as often. Don't be surprised if you no longer need to snack. Many people do well on 2 or 3 meals a day. If you need snacks:

Slices of cheese and ham rolled with a vegetable (some people eat cheese with butter) Oilseed

olives

(macadamias, walnuts, hazelnuts, cashews, etc.)

A piece of cheese

A boiled egg, kept in the refrigerator

Canned tuna

Olives and nuts can replace potato chips in front of the TV. If you're always hungry between meals, you're probably not eating enough fat. Don't be afraid of fat. Eat more fat until you feel full.

Dining out or meals with friends

Restaurants: generally not a big problem. You can ask to replace the potatoes with salad. For meat dishes, ask for extra butter.

Fast food: Kebab can be a decent option (preferably avoid bread). At burger chains, hamburger steaks are usually the least worst option. Avoid soda and chips, obviously. Drink water. Pizza toppings are generally ok, and the stricter you are, the less dough you'll eat.

If you eat strictly on a daily basis, it won't be a problem to make some exceptions when invited to eat out. If you're not sure what you'll be served, you can grab a bite to eat at home before heading out.

Nuts and cheeses are good "emergency foods" for when there are no other suitable options available

Shopping list for beginners

Print this list and take it to the bakery/supermarket/grocery store:

Butter

Sour cream (40% fat)

Sour cream (34% fat)

Eggs

Bacon

Meat (ground, steaks, cubes, fillets, etc.)

Fish (preferably fatty fish such as salmon and mackerel)

Cheese (preferably high fat)

Yogurt grevo (10% fat)

Cabbage, cauliflower, broccoli, Brussels sprouts

Other vegetables that grow above ground

Frozen vegetables

Avocados

Olives

Olive oil

Oilseeds

Clean out your pantry!

Want to maximize your chances of success? Especially if you have difficulty with cravings and sugar addiction, it is wise to throw away (or donate) sugary foods, starchy foods, "light" products, etc. Are included:

Candies

"Chips"

Soft drinks and juices

Margarines

Sugar in all forms

Bread

Pasta

Rice

Potatoes

Breakfast cereals

Everything that says "low fat" or "fat free"

Ice cream

Cookies

Why not do it now?

The serpent in paradise

Be very skeptical of "low-carb" products such as pasta or chocolate. Unfortunately, these products are often junk. They have prevented many people from losing weight, and are usually full of carbohydrates when you can look beyond the creative marketing.

For example, Dreamfileds "low carb pasta" is practically pure starch, and is absorbed in more or less the same way as any other pasta:

The Dreamfields pasta scam

How about low carb bread? Be careful: if it contains grains, it is certainly not low-carb. But some companies still try to sell it to you as a low carb option. Here is an example:

Fake Low Carb Bread from Julian Bakery

Low-carb chocolate is usually full of polyols ("sugar alcohols": xylitol, maltitol, etc.), which the manufacturer does not count as carbohydrates. But roughly speaking, half of these carbohydrates can be absorbed, increasing blood glucose and insulin. The rest of these carbs end up in the large intestine, potentially causing gas and diarrhea. Furthermore, any sweeteners can keep sugar cravings alive.

If you want to be healthy and slim, eat real food instead.

Revenues

Easy ways to prepare eggs:

Place the eggs in cold water and wait for them to boil. Leave 4 minutes for soft eggs, or 8 minutes for hard eggs. Eat them with mayonnaise (but read the ingredients first to make sure it works!) if you want.

Fry the eggs in butter on 1 or 2 sides. Season with salt and pepper.

Melt butter in a frying pan and add 2 eggs and 2-3 tablespoons of cream. Add salt and pepper. Stir until ready. Place spring onions and grated cheese on top. Serve with fried bacon.

Make an omelet with 3 eggs and 3 tablespoons of cream. Add salt and seasoning. Melt butter in the pan and pour the mixture over the top. When the omelet sets, you can top it with tasty things. For example, one or several types of cheese, fried bacon and mushrooms, good sausages (read the ingredients!) or even leftovers from last night's dinner. Fold the omelet in half and serve with a salad.

Instead of bread

Will it be difficult for you to give up bread? Ooopsies are a good option. It is a carbohydrate-free "bread" that can be eaten in several ways.

Oopsies

(makes 6 to 8, depending on size)

3 eggs

100g cream cheese

pinch of salt

½ teaspoon of psyllium or chia husks (optional)

½ teaspoon of chemical yeast (optional)

Separate the egg whites from the yolks

Beat the egg whites with salt until stiff. You should be able to turn the bowl upside down without the egg whites moving.

Mix the egg yolks and cream cheese well. If desired, add the psyllium/chia/yeast (this makes the oopsie more "bread-like")

Gently mix the egg whites with the egg yolk and cream cheese mixture – try to keep the air in the egg whites

Place 6 large or 8 small portions on a baking tray

Bake in the middle of the oven at 150°C for about 25 minutes – until they are golden brown.

You can eat oopsies as bread or use them to make sandwiches. You can also put different types of seeds in them before roasting them – for example: poppy, sesame or sunflower. A large oopsie can be used to make a Swiss roll: add a generous layer of whipped cream and some berries. Enjoy!

Less strict: some bread. Can't live without real bread? So eat a thin slice of bread and lots of butter and frosting. The more butter and add-ons, the less bread you will need to feel full.

Instead of potatoes, rice, pasta

Cauliflower puree: chop the cauliflower into small pieces and cook them with a pinch of salt, until they are soft. Remove the water. Add cream, butter, and knead.

Salads made from vegetables that grow above ground, perhaps with some type of cheese. Try different types of

Cooked broccoli, cauliflower or Brussels sprouts.

Vegetables au gratin: fry them in butter. Add salt and pepper. Place in a refractory and add grated cheese. Heat to 225°C, until the cheese melts and browns.

Cooked vegetables, with cream. For example, cabbage or spinach

"Cauliflower rice": grate the cauliflower; boil for 1 or 2 minutes. Great substitute for

Avocado rice

Snacks and desserts

Various oilseeds: macadamias, Brazil nuts, hazelnuts, walnuts…

Sausages: cut into pieces, and attach a piece of cheese with a toothpick

Vegetables with sauce: try cucumber "sticks", peppers (green, red and yellow), cauliflower, etc.

Cream cheese rolls: Roll cream cheese around thin slices of salami, ham or long strips of cucumber. LCHF

Olive

Chips: on a baking sheet, form small mounds of grated parmesan. Heat in the oven at 225°C. Let them melt and turn a beautiful color (be careful – they burn easily). Serve as chips, perhaps with some sauce.

THANKS

CLARE DOMINIC